The Acid Reflux Drink Recipe Book

100 Delicious Drinks to Prevent and Provide Relief from Acid Reflux, GERD and Heartburn

Amy Lyric

Table of Contents

Almond Butter Smoothie

Blueberry Bliss

Fruit-Loaded Smoothie

Green Aloe Vera Smoothie

Cantaloupe Chia Smoothie

Golden Beet Smoothie with Applesauce

Creamy Avocado & Raspberry Smoothie

BEFORE-MEAL JUICES

Apple and Kale Juice

Carrot, Apple, and Beet Juice

Green Mango Juice

Gingery Cabbage Pear Juice

Diluted Melon and Parsley Juice

Banana and Celery Juice

Watermelon and Basil Juice

Herbed Melony Juice

The Green Monster

Lettuce, Aloe Vera, and Avocado Juice

Papaya, Radish, and Cilantro Juice

Blueberry Juice with Cucumber and Chard

Spinach, Carrot, and Honeydew Juice

Orange Balancer

Peach and Ginger Juice

All-Fruit Juice

Rainbow Booster

Golden Beet and Fig Juice

Kale, Celery, and Cantaloupe Juice

Gingery Spinach, Fennel, and Mango Juice

COLD AFTERNOON REFRESHMENTS

Lavender Iced Drink

Cucumber Water

Very Berry Flavored Water

Chamomile and Ginger Iced Tea

Melon Infused Water

Ginger Ale

Rocking Ginger Apple Juice

Maple and Apple Iced Tea

Watermelon Water

Nettle Iced Tea

Gingery Iced Drink

Vanilla and Pear Water

Fuji Apple & Cinnamon Iced Drink

Apple Cider

Hibiscus Iced Drink

Peach Iced Tea

Blackberry & Rosemary Infused Water

Rocking Aloe Vera Juice with Figs

SPECIAL EVENT DRINKS

Peach Cream "Soda"

Rosemary-Flavored Ginger & Apple Mimosas

Honeydew & Ginger "Spritzer"

Mango Raspberry Ice Cream Shaker

Lavender Blueberry "Spritzer"

Red & Orange Mocktail

Cucumber "Mojito"

Peach Apple Shake

Sugary Peach Apple Cider

Grilled Papaya & Pear Mocktail

A Different Shirley Temple

Watermelon Ginger Cooler

Virgin Mai Tai

Cucumber Fig Cooler

Tropical Cheesecake Mocktail

WARMING & RELIEVING TEA

CONCLUSION

Introduction

Sentenced to a life without coffee? Or champagne at your promotion party? Or even a glass of lemonade to beat the heat on a summer afternoon? I know it sounds like the end of the world, but once you stop seeing your new restrictive diet as a challenge, and sign up for a fun and adventurous ride, you will not only learn that mojitos are overrated but that the fruit and vegetable combos you can explore are pretty endless, as well.

And that's exactly what this book offers – a fun and highly enjoyable journey that will show you that heartburn and acid reflux are not to be feared but tamed.

If some (or most) of your days are disrupted by sharp and painful burning sensations in your chest, then it is about time you found a way to put a stop to it. Fortunately, this book was made to help you with just that – to find a non-overwhelming way to replenish your tummy acids without sacrificing your taste buds. And while you can find tons of heartburn-relieving meal recipes online, when it comes to beverages, there is pretty much zero advice out there that goes beyond yogurt and tea. I say it's about time we changed that.

Enriching your heartburn-friendly recipe folder with 100 irresistible drink recipes that are highly alkalizing, soothing, and balancing, **this book will help you restore the balance in your gut in no time.**

From helping you to recognize and approach your unique condition, to providing you with the most detailed list of foods that should be privileged or avoided by the heartburn sufferer, this book is the only guide for knocking down heartburn you will ever need.

Whether you are in a mood for:

- *A morning smoothie*
- *A yummy juice before dinner*
- *A cold refreshing beverage*
- *A mocktail*
- *The perfect cup of tea to warm and ease your tummy with*

this book will definitely come as a reward.

And who doesn't like rewards? Jump to the first chapter and see how you can claim yours!

Explaining the Corrosive Condition

Call it GERD, heartburn, acid reflux, or simply indigestion, you are probably explaining the same thing – a painful burning sensation behind your breastbone. But do all of these terms actually refer to the same condition? Well, yes and no.

Although they are all connected and often used interchangeably, GERD, acid reflux, and heartburn actually represent different things. Whether you are suffering from occasional heartburn or a chronic GERD, the symptoms are pretty much the same. However, knowing exactly what these terms represent can help you battle your condition and knock down that painfully irritating burning sensation.

Heartburn

If your grandma used to recommend baking soda for the irritating pain in your chest, she was most likely right – it was heartburn. Heartburn – as misleading as it sounds - actually happens in the digestive tract. When your stomach lining is thinner than the lining of your esophagus (also known as *the food pipe*), the acid from the esophagus causes a painful, burning, and tightening sensation in your chest.

Heartburn usually occurs right after eating and it is a common condition that millions of people experience every single day.

Acid Reflux

Acid Reflux is what actually causes the heartburn. Your stomach has a circular muscle called LES (Lower Esophageal Sphincter). After the consumed food passes through the food pipe and goes into your stomach, the job of the LES is to tighten the food pipe. In a normal cycle of digestion, this works as a one-way valve. The food tube allows the food to pass into the stomach, while at the same time blocking the contents of the stomach from flowing back up.

When the LES muscle is weakened and fails to do its job efficiently, the not-properly-tightened esophagus allows the acids from the stomach to move backward and enter the food pipe. This is known as acid reflux and this condition not only causes heartburn but a number of other irritating symptoms such as sore throat and coughing.

GERD

Like I said, heartburn is a common occurrence and this burning sensation shouldn't be a warning sign if it is experienced every now and then after a rich meal. But, if heartburn occurs more than two or three times a week, this is usually a clear sign that you suffer from GERD.

GERD or Gastroesophageal Reflux Disease is a frequent acid reflux and it is commonly described as *chronic heartburn.*

When the stomach acid frequently moves back to the esophagus, the acid reflux can seriously irritate the lining of your food pipe. This causes inflammation of the esophagus which is known as GERD.

The severity of this condition depends on the degree of the dysfunction of the LES, the type (as well as the amount) of the fluid that is moved backward to the food pipe, as well as the saliva's neutralizing effect.

What If It Is Chronic?

Although frequent heartburn is the most common sign of this condition, GERD has a number of other symptoms that you need to watch out for. Here is the list of the symptoms that GERD sufferers most commonly experience:

- Frequent Heartburn
- Bad Breath
- Chest Pain
- Persistent Dry Cough
- Trouble Swallowing
- Tooth Enamel Damage (which happens as a result of excess acid)
- Asthma
- Regurgitation

Whilst can you easily self-diagnose with this list of symptoms, if your pay a visit to your doctor which is recommended, they will probably prescribe a test to confirm the GERD diagnosis and check for possible complications. The most common tests for diagnosing GERD are:

- *Esophageal Manometry* – measuring the esophagus' muscle contractions when swallowing.

- *Upper Endoscopy* – a thin tube with a camera attached is inserted down the throat to examine the esophagus.

- *Ambulatory Acid (pH) Probe Test* – a monitor place in the food pipe identifies the acid regularities that occur there.

- *Upper Digestive System X-Ray* – an x-ray is taken after drinking chalky beverage that coats the insides of the digestive tract.

Who Is at Risk?

GERD makes no discrimination. It can affect everyone from infants to seniors. The reason why this condition happens is the LES malfunctioning. But why does the LES malfunction in the first place?

Many different reasons can contribute to the weakening of this muscle so you will have to do a full examination with your doctor to pinpoint exactly what causes the irregularities in your digestive tract.

Although they vary from person to person, the most common causes of GERD are:

- Smoking
- Frequent Alcohol Consumption
- Being Overweight or Obese
- Pregnancy
- Hiatal Hernia
- Connective Tissue Disorders
- Certain LES weakening medicines such as calcium channel blockers, antihistamines, sedatives, etc.

The Dangers Behind This Condition

Although the term *chronic* may send chills down your spine, GERD is actually a condition that is easily manageable and can be treated with simple lifestyle and dietary modifications. When changes are made, that is. If left untreated, the inflammation of your esophagus can cause:

- *Esophageal Stricture* – Formation of a scar tissue that narrows the food pipe and results in problems with swallowing.

- *Esophageal Ulcer* – Formation of open sore in the food pipe that can result in bleeding and extremely painful swallowing.

- *Barret's Esophagus* – Changes in the food pipe's tissue that increases the risk of developing esophageal cancer.

The Acid Reflux Diet Makeover

Admit it! You can name at least three foods that spell trouble for that awful burning sensation in your chest. So why are they still in your fridge? Revamping your diet is the first and most important step that you need to take towards a reflux-reduced life. And the best part? You'd be surprised to know that even the simple dietary tweaks can make you feel significantly better.

Since acid reflux is a digestive disease, it is understandable that foods are the biggest triggers for the unwanted symptoms. Sacrificing your guilty pleasures may seem like a boring way to eat your dinner, go to a party, or even watch a movie without your favorite snack, but the health results will be tremendous. I promise, once your acid reflux is tamed, all will have been worth it.

Healthifying Your Kitchen

It is common for acid reflux and GERD sufferers to experience heartburn and painful sensations after eating a meal. But do you know what part of the meal is actually causing your chest to burn? Is it the meat? The spices? A certain veggie? The way in which the dish is prepared? Your painful symptoms may not be triggered by your favorite meal but by a single ingredient in the dish. And who knows? Maybe it isn't the hamburger itself that is causing you heartburn. Maybe it is the fact that it has raw onions in it.

That is why it is of utmost importance for you to know the types of foods that shouldn't be included in your diet, so you can mix and match healthy ingredients and find the best way for you to satisfy your taste buds without feeling the pain behind your breastbone.

Beware the "C" Triggers

The first group of foods that you absolutely need to purge from your diet (and hopefully your kitchen) is the "C" triggers. Obviously, not everything that starts with a "C" should be avoided (think carrot), however, clumping the "C" triggers in a single category will help you remember not to include these foods in your diet:

Caffeine. If a double latte is your best friend, you will absolutely hate the fact that coffee has no place in the acid reflux diet. Caffeine is known to weaken the LES and forces the stomach to generate even more acids, which is definitely not a good news if your food pipe is inflamed. Besides, caffeine also negatively affects GABA (a substance that is crucial for the balance in the digestive tract), which is yet another reason why you should switch to tea instead, as long as it is free of caffeine.

And in case you were wondering, the decaf latte will do you just as much trouble as the caffeinated kind. It is actually the oil in the coffee beans (both decaf and caffeinated) that aggravate the acid reflux, so the decaf cup of coffee is not your friend either.

Citrus. You don't need to be a nutritionist to know that citrus fruits contain tons of citric acid. Consuming foods with high acidity will further complicate your already vexing condition, so make sure that lemons, limes, oranges, and other citrus fruits are avoided. Even people that do not have acid reflux can experience discomfort after consuming a citrus fruit; that's how negatively these fruits can affect the digestive tract. You can only imagine how strong the intensity of the heartburn can be if your gut is vulnerable to it.

This includes eating, juicing, or even diluting citrus fruit with water. Even a teaspoon of the juice mixed in a smoothie can affect your acid reflux negatively. Yes, they may be healthy and they may be jam-packed with vitamins, but citrus fruits are simply not for you.

Chocolate

Unfortunately for you, chocolate is also a trigger. I know that there isn't better comfort food than chocolate, but the caffeine in the chocolate can also trigger your reflux. Besides, chocolate also contains *theobromine* (a stimulant that can cause heartburn).

But that's not the main reason why you should rethink swallowing a chocolate cupcake. Its main ingredient, cocoa, has been scientifically proven to aggravate reflux. Another reason is that of its feel-good properties. The serotonin in the chocolate – which is known to be relaxing – also relaxes the LES. And since we know that the job of the LES is to tighten up not to relax, you can see how wrong this is for your acid reflux, not to mention GERD.

Need to take your sugar fix? Switch to dark chocolate, white chocolate, and ideally – eat some sweet fruit.

Canned Foods. No, canned foods are not on this list because fresh ingredients are far healthier and more nutritious (although that is something you need to keep in mind). Canned foods are not a good choice for those prone to heartburn because they trigger the burning and painful symptoms. How? Canned foods are more acidic than the fresh produce. They are pumped up with acidity so that their shell life is increased, as well as to kill the bacteria inside the can. And since acidity is not something you need in your food pipe, rethink buying foods in cans.

Carbonated Drinks. I will not waste your time explaining the side effects of drinking soda because pretty much everyone is well aware of this one. What I want to focus on is sparkling water. There is a huge controversy wrapped around whether sparkling water is good for the heartburn or not, so I want to clear this confusion once and for all.

Carbonated water increases the pressure inside your stomach which contributes to the malfunction of your LES. The carbonation in the sparkling water increases the stomach distension. For instance, if you drink a pint of regular water, your stomach will, obviously, distend only by a pint. But, if you drink a pint of sparkling water, your stomach will distend twice as much. Now, you may think that burping relieves your heartburn symptoms, but this is not true. All that the bubbles in this fuzzy drink can do is relax the lower opening of your food pipe and allow the stomach acid to creep up the gullet.

Although not so severe, other "C" triggers that you need to avoid are *cranberries* and *cherries.*

Other Culprits to Avoid
Here are the types of foods that should never be on your dinner table:

Fatty Foods. Whether we are talking about greasy potato fries or grilled fatty meat, if the food has a high fat content, it is best not to consume it. Foods that are high in fat content stay in the stomach longer, which, obviously, forces our stomach to produce more stomach acid. And since, at the same time, the fatty foods cause the LES to relax, this will only cause more stomach acid to enter your esophagus.

That being said, try to avoid eating meat, or if you cannot give up the occasional steak, stick to the lean cuts of meat only. Also, do not choose whole dairy products.

Alcohol. Even a single glass of your favorite alcoholic beverage can backfire in a lot of ways for the acid reflux sufferer. People seem to find excuses to enjoy a fun evening out such as *Alcohol doesn't have acidity so my reflux will be fine.* However, it is not the acidity that aggravates the reflux. Alcohol actually makes it more difficult for the body to clear the piled up acid from the food pipe, and that is what aggravates your symptoms. Besides, alcohol is also known to cause damage to the sensitive esophagus, so there is yet another reason for you to sip on a non-alcoholic beverage instead.

Certain Spices. Many of the spices that are commonly used to improve the meal flavor are actually reflux triggers. The most common spices that cause heartburn are:

- Chili Powder
- Curry Powder
- Mustard
- Pepper (Black, Cayenne, White, Red)
- Nutmeg

But just because some people who have frequent heartburns find nutmeg to be a trigger doesn't mean that it also cause heartburn to you. It is trickier to discover which spice is a trigger and which isn't since they are not consumed on their own, however, there is a rule that fresh is always better. It is unlikely for fresh herbs to aggravate reflux so feel free to give flavor and aroma to your meals and drinks that way.

The only exception to the "fresh is better" rule is **mint**. Mint can freshen your breath and give your drinks a refreshing taste, however, it can also inflame your acid reflux by allowing the LES to relax and making it easy for stomach acids to flow backward.

Tomatoes. For people who suffer from acid reflux - or even worse, GERD - tomatoes can have a negative impact on their health. Due to their high acidity content, tomatoes can be a real irritant for your food pipe. They inflame the lining of the esophagus and aggravate the reflux symptoms. Whether raw or in a sauce, it is best to skip the meals that contain tomatoes for the sake of your tummy.

Raw Onions. For those that rarely experience heartburn, is it not likely that eating raw onions will result in any burning sensation. But, if the irritating pain in your chest is known to disrupt most of your days, onions may not be such a good choice for you. It is proven that raw onions are not friendly for the sensitive esophagus so make sure not to include them in your meals and salads.

Raw Garlic. Although there are many conflicting theories when it comes to the relationship of garlic and acid reflux, it is best to avoid raw garlic. Cooked garlic is safe to eat and may even reduce the reflux symptoms according to some nutritionists, but the raw kind can do the opposite.

pH – Why Does It Matter?

I don't know about you, but when someone mentions the pH value, the first thing that comes to my mind is *shampoo*. Maybe that is because of their annoying commercials or the fact that pretty much every shampoo has "pH balanced" written all over the label. Be as it may, advertising the balanced pH is a clear indicator that the product contains the ideal pH value. However, when you suffer from acid reflux, looking for the perfect pH balance in the food that goes into your stomach is far more important than buying the right product to wash your hair with.

But what is the pH value, and why does it matter? The pH scale measures the acidity and the alkalinity of the foods. For those who have a very sensitive food pipe, the pH scale is super important as they need to strive to include foods that are low in acidity.

Low in acidity means high in alkalinity and the other way around. That being said, you need to make sure that your diet is packed with alkaline foods and lacks the acid ones.

The scale of the pH values can get somewhat confusing, so let me simplify this. The scale ranges from 0 to 14. A pH of 0 means totally acidic and a pH of 14 means completely alkaline. A pH of 7 is neutral (or balanced like in those shampoos I mentioned earlier). Water has pH of 7 and is completely neutral. But don't let this confuse you, you cannot eat foods with pH of 14. Outside the human body, foods have pH that is lower than 7. Alkaline foods are those that are closer to a pH of 7.

Want to know which veggies and fruits are the safest for the acid reflux sufferers to consume? Here are their pH values:

VEGETABLES

Type of Veggie	pH Value
Asparagus	6
Beets	5.3 – 6.5
Broccoli	6.3 – 6.5
Brussels Sprouts	6 – 6.3
Cabbage	5.2 – 6.8
Carrots	5.8 – 6.4
Cauliflower	5.6
Celery	5.7 – 6
Corn	5.9 – 7.3
Cucumbers	5.1 – 5.8
Eggplant	5.5 – 6.5
Garlic	5.8

Ginger	5.6 – 5.9
Kale	6.4 – 6.8
Leeks	5.5 – 6.1
Lettuce	5.8 – 6.1
Parsley (although a herb)	5.7 – 6
Peas	6.4 – 6.8
Peppers	5.2 – 5.9
Potatoes	5.4 – 5.9
Radishes	5.8 – 6
Spinach	5.5 – 6.8
Squash	5.8 – 6
Swiss Chard	6.2 – 6.8
Tomatoes	4.3 – 4.8
Turnips	5.3 – 5.9
Yams	5.5 – 6.8
Zucchini	5.7 – 6.1

FRUITS

Type of Fruit	pH Value
Apples	3.9
Apricots	3.3 – 3.5
Avocados	6.3 – 6.6
Bananas	5 – 5.3
Blueberries	3.2
Cantaloupe	6.1 – 6.6
Figs	5 – 5.9
Grapes	3 – 3.5
Grapefruit	3 – 3.3
Lemon Juice	2 – 2.9
Mango	5.8 – 6
Melons	6 – 6.7
Nectarines	3.9 – 4.2
Orange Juice	3.3 – 4
Papaya	6.7
Peaches	3.3 – 4
Pears	3.5 – 4.6
Pineapple	3.2 – 4
Plums	3.4
Pomegranate	2.9 – 3.2
Prunes	3.6 – 4.3
Raspberries	3.2 – 3.9
Strawberries	3 – 3.9
Tangerine	3.3 – 4
Watermelon	5.2 – 5.6

Reflux-Fighting Foods to Consume

Although non-acidic foods are all generally safe to consume, there are certain types of foods that can lower the GERD symptoms, knock down the acid reflux, and bring balance back to your tummy by relieving it from the corrosive heartburn. Such foods include:

Ginger – When consumed in moderation, ginger can be a strong weapon against esophagus' inflammation and heartburn. Make ginger tea, include in juices and cold beverages, grate into sauces and soups and enjoy its powerful flavor and aroma.

Aloe Vera – A powerful antioxidant and a natural healing agent that can help you lower the reflux symptoms in no time. You can either purchase it as a whole plant or find the leaves and liquid separately in most well-equipped health-food stores.

Yogurt - Thanks to its probiotic properties, yogurt is one of the best foods to consume when trying to eat and drink your way to a heartburn-free gut. It is creamy, delicious, plus it helps you fight the acid reflux. What's not to like? Just make sure to stick to the low-fat and unsweetened varieties and watch your heartburn disappear.

Oatmeal - Your breakfast favorite is not only allowed on your special tummy-healthy diet but also recommended. Oatmeal is packed with fiber which is great for reducing your reflux symptoms and absorbing the stomach acids.

Speaking of fiber, whole grain rice and whole grain bread are also great for fighting your acid reflux. Their thick texture can coat the lining of your stomach and relieve the symptoms significantly, so make sure to incorporate them into your diet.

Banana – It is a no-brainer that highly acidic foods can worsen your symptoms and should be avoided. Foods that are highly alkaline, on the other hand, can help neutralize the acids in your stomach and restore the balance. And bananas, thanks to their high pH value, are one of those foods.

Green Veggies – There isn't a dietary plan that doesn't include green veggies, and the acid reflux diet is no exception either. Green vegetables, especially leafy greens such as spinach and kale, are highly alkaline and can be a powerful weapon in knocking down heartburn. Incorporating them into your juices, smoothies, and salads, is a perfect way to boost your tummy balance.

Melon. Whether we are talking about honeydew, watermelon, or cantaloupe, blending melon into your smoothies can also have a positive impact on your condition. Highly alkaline and great in keeping the stomach acid balanced, these fruits can help you keep the acid reflux at bay.

Fennel. If you like the taste of this mildly-licorice-flavored veggie, then it can make a significant improvement for your super-sensitive food pipe. Thanks to its highly alkaline properties, fennel is known to improve the stomach function by balancing its acids.

Avocado. Technically, avocado is loaded with fat. But the fatty content of this green fruit will not put more stress on your already sensitive tummy. Quite the contrary. The healthy monounsaturated fats that avocados are packed with will not only lower your cholesterol levels but also support the elimination of the acid reflux symptoms. Just be careful when eating guacamole as it is often made with heartburn-unfriendly ingredients such as onions, lime, and garlic.

Parsley. Did you know that parsley is one of the most powerful natural remedies that fight indigestion? And if that's not enough for you to sneak this lovely herb into your juices, smoothies, and salads, then perhaps this will change your mind – parsley is also great at soothing the throat which is mainly why it is so helpful for those suffering from GERD and acid reflux. Add a handful of parsley and say farewell to your dry cough.

Licorice Root. When it comes to making medicine, licorice used is a very popular and commonly used ingredient. And the best part? Licorice root is great for treating digestive issues such as indigestion, heartburn, and stomach inflammation. It is also very successful in soothing the throat, which is yet another reason why you should include it in your diet. Buy licorice root in a well-equipped health-food store and make yourself a cup of warming licorice tea for a healthy gut.

Drinking Your Way to Balanced Tummy

It doesn't matter if you are suffering from acid reflux, GERD, or even have an occasional heartburn. Despite of the severity your condition, if heartburn is a familiar occurrence for you, then you probably know how most drinks only add fuel to the fire burning behind your breastbone. And even when you are paying attention and avoiding the triggers, it seems kind of impossible to say farewell to all the yummy stuff.

But just because your favorites are not allowed, it doesn't mean that you cannot create fun and super delicious beverages that will not only satisfy your tummy, but it will also balance its acids and restore the pH balance.

The Art of Making Easing Beverages

Yes, I call it an *art*. Of course you will fail if you look at the process of consuming heartburn-friendly foods an overwhelming challenge. You need to shift your point of view from a restrictive to a fun and rewarding experience.

How can you possibly live without coffee? Or green tea? Or soda? Or mojitos? What will you drink at parties? What will you serve when hosting an event? How to refresh yourself when mint and lemonade are no longer an option? I know how hard may this challenge seem to you, but once you determine to make the most of it, you will see that all of these things are pretty overrated.

Herbal Tea

One of the most beneficial thing for your tummy is a cup of warming and soothing tea. From ginger, licorice, chamomile, nettle, to more advanced options such as barley, rooibos, and elderflower, tea can be number one weapon against that painful sensation behind your breastbone.

But who says that drinking tea is no fun? If you are not a tea fan or do not enjoy drinking non-caffeinated tea, you can easily spice things up with your favorite ingredients. Here is how you can do that:

- Add dried fruits to your tea. This will not only infuse the flavor but it will also add additional health benefits to your warming cup.
- Add aromatics such as ginger, vanilla, cinnamon, or whatever your taste buds find pleasing. As long as it is acid reflux friendly, of course.
- Sweeten it up. Adding maples syrup to your cup of tea is a great way to improve the taste and make it much more enjoyable.

- Vary it. If you don't like the taste, make it different and see what suits you. Other than the tips above, you can also improve the taste by adding a tablespoon of fruit juice or even a splash of milk.

This book offers eighteen different ways to prepare delicious, warming, and easing teas.

Smoothies

Smoothies are a great – and probably the easiest – way to get the important nutrients without any hassle. Do you find some of the most beneficial ingredients awful? Incorporate them in smoothies along with sweet and pleasant ingredients. That way you will not even notice their unpleasant taste (think fennel) but still receive their benefits. How great is that?

This book rewards you with twenty morning smoothies that are filling, yummy and relieving.

Juices

Similar to smoothies, juices are also a great way to mix and match pleasant and unpleasant ingredients in order to pack your tummy with the healthiest and most soothing ingredients.

In the section called "Before Meal Juices" I will provide you with 20 different juice recipes that you can enjoy about 60 – 30 minutes before your meals. By doing so, you will allow your gut to begin the process of digestion earlier in order to tolerate your meals better. Besides, drinking juices before meal will allow you to fill your tummy a bit so you will not be so hungry. This will prevent you from overeating, which as you know, is hazardous for your condition.

Be creative when making juices as well. If your juice is too creamy, dilute it with some water for even better digestion.

Fancy Drinks

You don't have to avoid parties or hosting events just because you cannot enjoy a traditional cocktail. There are many different ways in which you can enjoy delicious and elegant-looking drinks, and decrease your acid reflux symptoms at the same time.

There are plenty of healthy and delicious ingredients that your acid reflux totally approves of, and if you know how to mix them properly, you will never miss an alcoholic and bubbly drink ever again.

In the section called "Special Event Drinks" you will find 24 fancy and delicious mocktails to serve at your next event. And the best part? Each and every one of these heartburn-friendly cocktails will support your gut health.

Other Beverages

There are many other ways in which you can sneak in the benefits of the healthiest acid reflux relieving ingredients. Iced tea and infused water are just some of the many.

Iced tea is a great way to combine both tea and healthy fruits and herbs, and infused water is excellent if you need to trick yourself into drinking more water. Check out the section called "Cold Afternoon Refreshments" and see the delightfully refreshing recipes that can help you keep heartburn at bay.

Energizing Morning Smoothies

Please note that these smoothies are not supposed to replace your hearty breakfast. They should be consumed in addition to a balanced and healthy morning meal with the purpose of adding an additional energy kick and restoring the balance in your tummy.

Those smoothies that contain oats or almond flour are an exception as they can make a healthy and balancing breakfast.

Banana & Oat Smoothie

Packed with three highly alkaline ingredients, this smoothie is great for balancing your stomach acids in the morning.

Serves: 1

Ready in: 5 minutes

Ingredients:

1 Banana
½ Avocado
2/3 cup Almond Milk
¼ cup Instant Oats
¼ tsp Vanilla Extract

Preparation:

1. Place all of the ingredients in the bowl of your blender.
2. Blend for about a minute or so, until really smooth.
3. Serve immediately and enjoy!

Green Yogurt Kick

The probiotics in the yogurt and the alkaline properties in the other ingredient will give you a nice morning kick that will destroy your heartburn in a jiffy.

Serves: 1

Ready in: 5 minutes

Ingredients:

½ Gala Apple
½ cup Spinach
½ Banana
¾ cup Yogurt
¼ cup cubed Papaya

Preparation:

1. Peel and core the apple and then chop it into smaller pieces.
2. Place the apple along with the other ingredients in the bowl of your blender.
3. Blend for a minute, or until smooth.
4. Serve immediately and enjoy.

Sweet Red Kefir

Packed with probiotics from the kefir and balancing alkaline compounds from the beets and bananas, this smoothie will balance and energize your morning. Add a dash of cinnamon for some extra flavor.

Serves: 2

Ready in: 5 minutes

Ingredients:

1 Banana
1 cup peeled and cubed Beets
1 cup Kefir
1 ½ tbsp Maple Syrup

Preparation:

1. Place all of the ingredients in your blender.
2. Blend for a minute or two, or until smooth.
3. Pour into 2 serving glasses.
4. Consume immediately and enjoy!

Avocado and Frozen Banana Smoothie

You can substitute the frozen bananas with regular bananas and a few cubes of ice, but keep in mind that ice will dilute the flavor. Make sure not to use more than ½ cup of grapes as they are not that alkaline.

<u>*Serves:*</u> *1*

<u>*Ready in:*</u> *5 minutes*

Ingredients:

1 ½ Frozen Bananas
1 Avocado
½ cup Red Grapes
2 tbsp ground Almonds
1 ¼ cup Almond Milk
Pinch of Cinnamon

Preparation:

1. Peel the avocado and remove the pit.
2. Place it in the bowl of your blender along with the other ingredients.
3. Blend until smooth, about a minute or two.
4. Serve immediately and enjoy!

Carrot and Spinach Smoothie

The spinach and carrot will do wonders for your tummy. If the taste is too bland for your liking, add a tablespoon of maple syrup to sweeten it up.

Serves: 1

Ready in: 5 minutes

Ingredients:

1 large Carrot, chopped
1 Pear, peeled and chopped
1 cup Baby Spinach
¾ cup Coconut Water
¼ Avocado

Preparation:

1. Place all of the ingredients in the bowl of your blender.
2. Blend for a minute or until smooth.
3. Serve immediately and enjoy!

Tropical Smoothie

The coconut water in this smoothie will bring you relief from the acid reflux symptoms and help you start your day the right way.

<u>*Serves:*</u> 2

<u>*Ready in:*</u> *5 minutes*

Ingredients:

2 tbsp Coconut Flakes, unsweetened
1 Mango, peeled and chopped
½ cup Papaya Chunks
1 Banana
1 ¼ cup Coconut Water

Preparation:

1. Place all of the ingredients in the bowl of your blender.
2. Blend for a minute or until really smooth.
3. Pour into two glasses and serve immediately.
4. Enjoy!

Peachy and Gingery Balancer

Ginger, peach, and yogurt will balance the acids in your stomach with their powerful alkalizing properties. The maple syrup makes this smoothie taste like dessert.

Serves: 1

Ready in: 5 minutes

Ingredients:

1 Peach, chopped
½ cup Yogurt
¼ tsp grated Ginger
1 tbsp Maple Syrup
½ Apple (make sure to use sweet apples only as sour ones can only aggravate your sensitive gut)

Preparation:

1. Peel, core, and chop the apple.
2. Place it in the bowl of your blender along with the remaining ingredients.
3. Blend until smooth.
4. Serve immediately and enjoy!

Watermelon and Kale Smoothie

Highly alkaline, this smoothie will give you a balanced and energizing start of the day.

Serves: 1

Ready in: 5 minutes

Ingredients:

½ cup Watermelon Chunks
½ cup Kale
½ cup Vanilla Yogurt
Pinch of Ginger Powder

Preparation:

1. Place all of the ingredients in your blender.
2. Blend for a minute, until really smooth.
3. Pour into a serving glass and enjoy!

Melony Probiotic

Melon and kefir star in this heartburn-relieving recipe that will prepare you for starting your day without the irritating acid reflux symptoms.

Serves: 2

Ready in: 5 minutes

Ingredients:

1 cup Kefir
1 cup Melon Chunks
1 tsp minced Ginger
A handful of Watercress
½ Cucumber

Preparation:

1. Peel and chop the cucumber and place it in your blender along with the remaining ingredients.
2. Blend until the mixture becomes smooth.
3. Serve immediately and enjoy!

Dandelion and Fig Smoothie

The dandelion greens are great in balancing the pH. If you do not like figs, you can use other alkaline fruits instead.

<u>*Serves:*</u> 1

<u>*Ready in:*</u> *5 minutes*

Ingredients:

2 Figs
1/2 cup Dandelion Greens
A handful of Spinach
½ cup Yogurt
¼ tsp grated Ginger

Preparation:

1. Place all of the ingredients in your blender.
2. Blend until the mixture becomes smooth, about a minute.
3. Serve immediately and enjoy!

Banana Peanut Butter Smoothie

Apple, banana, peanut butter, and milk is not just a delicious combination. It is also one that will bring balance back to your tummy.

Serves: 2

Ready in: 5 minutes

Ingredients:

2 tbsp Peanut Butter
2 Bananas
1 Sweet Apple
2/3 cup Milk
¼ tsp Vanilla Extract

Preparation:

1. Peel, core, and chop the apple.
2. Place it in the bowl of your blender along with the remaining ingredients.
3. Blend until smooth.
4. Pour into two glasses and enjoy!

Green Weapon

This powerful combination of alkalizing greens and mango will support your tummy health and prepare for a heartburn-free day.

Serves: 1

Ready in: 5 minutes

Ingredients:

½ cup Baby Spinach
2 Kale Leaves, chopped
A handful of Watercress
1 Mango, chopped
½ cup Coconut Water
½ Sweet Apple

Preparation:

1. Peel, core, and chop the apple.
2. Place it in your blender along with the remaining ingredients.
3. Blend until the mixture becomes smooth.
4. Serve immediately and enjoy!

Honeydew Reliever

Honeydew, oats, and avocado pack this smoothie with alkalizing properties that your stomach craves. If you want it to be less creamy, substitute the avocado for a non-creamy alkaline fruit.

Serves: 2

Ready in: 5 minutes

Ingredients:

1 cup Honeydew Chunks
¼ Avocado
2 tbsp Instant Oats
½ cup Milk
1 tbsp Maple Syrup
¼ tsp Vanilla Extract

Preparation:

1. Place all of the ingredients in the bowl of your blender.
2. Blend until the mixture becomes smooth.
3. Serves immediately and enjoy!

Almond Butter Smoothie

The creaminess of the almond butter and avocado make this smoothie a very enjoyable drink that your tummy will certainly benefit from.

Serves: 1

Ready in: 5 minutes

Ingredients:

½ cup Almond Milk
1 tbsp Almond Butter
½ Avocado
1 Pear
Pinch of Cinnamon

Preparation:

1. Peel, core, and chop the pear.
2. Place it in your blender along with the remaining ingredients.
3. Blend for a minute, or until smooth.
4. Serve immediately and enjoy!

Blueberry Bliss

Berries are not exactly highly recommended for those with acid reflux or GERD, but they are also not that harmful so avoiding their anti-inflammatory properties completely is not suggested. As long as you combine them with alkaline ingredients, your belly should stay balanced.

<u>*Serves:*</u> *1*

<u>*Ready in:*</u> *5 minutes*

Ingredients:

¼ cup Blueberries
2/3 cup Yogurt
1 tbsp Applesauce (made with sweet apples), unsweetened
Pinch of Cinnamon

Preparation:

1. Place all of the ingredients in the bowl of your blender.
2. Blend the mixture until smooth.
3. Pour into a serving glass immediately.
4. Enjoy!

Fruit-Loaded Smoothie

A bunch of alkaline fruits star in this recipe and will pack your mornings with tummy-soothing properties.

Serves: 2

Ready in: 5 minutes

Ingredients:

½ cup Watermelon Chunks
1 Pear, peeled and chopped
1 Mango, peeled and chopped
1 large Fig
1 cup Coconut Water

Preparation:

1. Place the watermelon, pear, mango, and fig, in the bowl of your blender.
2. Pour the coconut water over and put the lid on.
3. Blend until smooth.
4. Serve immediately and enjoy!

Green Aloe Vera Smoothie

The detoxifying aloe vera juice combined with the alkaline greens will be a true healing bomb for your stomach. If you don't have the juice, you can just use the plant and plain or coconut water instead.

Serves: 1

Ready in: 5 minutes

Ingredients:

½ cup Aloe Vera Juice
1 cup Baby Spinach
½ cup chopped Collard Greens
1 Celery Stalk
1 Sweet Apple
1 tbsp Maple Syrup, optional

Preparation:

1. Place all of the ingredients in the bowl of your blender.
2. Blend for about a minute or until the mixture becomes smooth.
3. Pour into a serving glass and enjoy immediately.

Cantaloupe Chia Smoothie

Packed with the healthiest ingredients for your gut, this smoothie will not only fill your tummy and balance its acids, but it will also satisfy your taste buds.

Serves: 2

Ready in: 5 minutes

Ingredients:

1 cup Cantaloupe Chunks
2 tbsp Chia Seeds
1 cup Yogurt
1 Apple

Preparation:

1. Peel, core, and chop the apple.
2. Place it in a blender and add the remaining ingredients.
3. Put the lid on and blend until it becomes smooth.
4. Serve immediately and enjoy!

Golden Beet Smoothie with Applesauce

This recipe uses kefir but you can use yogurt instead, if you want to. The probiotics from the kefir/yogurt really make all the difference here, so make sure not to use water.

Serves: 1

Ready in: 5 minutes

Ingredients:

½ cup chopped Golden Beets
2 tbsp Applesauce, unsweetened
½ cup Kefir
1 tbsp Maple Syrup
2 tbsp chopped Basil

Preparation:

1. Place all of the ingredients in your blender.
2. Blend for two minutes, or until smooth.
3. Pour into a serving glass.
4. Enjoy!

Creamy Avocado & Raspberry Smoothie

Raspberries may not be best when eaten in high quantities and on their own, but combined with avocado and ginger, they can really do magic for your vexing condition.

Serves: 3

Ready in: 5 minutes

Ingredients:

½ cup Raspberries
1 ½ Avocados
1 ½ tsp minced Ginger
½ Banana
½ cup Yogurt
½ cup Coconut Water

Preparation:

1. Scoop the flash out of the avocados and place in a blender.
2. Add the remaining ingredients and put the lid on.
3. Blend until smooth.
4. Pour into three serving glasses and enjoy!

Before-Meal Juices

To receive the benefits of these juices, it is best to consume them about 60 – 30 minutes before your meals. That will kick-start the digestion process and will help your gut digest your meal much more efficiently, which will, in turn, reduce the acid reflux symptoms.

All of these recipes, ideally require a juicer. If you don't own one, you can prepare them in your blender, instead. Of course, prepared in your blender they are technically smoothies, but if you strain them through a cheesecloth you will get clearer beverages similar to what the juicers offer.

Apple and Kale Juice

Packed with anti-inflammatory properties, this green juice will heal your gut and support digestion.

Serves: 2

Ready in: 5 minutes

Ingredients:

2 Large Apples, cut into eights
1 cup chopped Kale Leaves

Preparation:

1. Run all of the ingredients through your juicer.
2. Pour into two glasses.
3. Serve immediately and enjoy!

Carrot, Apple, and Beet Juice

Rich in some of the healthiest ingredients, this juice is perfect when consumed prior your meals. It will fill your tummy and support digestion.

Serves: 2

Ready in: 5 minutes

Ingredients:

1 Large Carrot
2 Large Sweet Apples, cut into eights
1 Beetroot, peeled and quartered
½ cup Spinach

Preparation:

1. Juice all of the ingredients following the instruction of your manufacturer.
2. Pour into two glasses.
3. Enjoy immediately!

Green Mango Juice

Collard greens, mango, and apple, make this juice great at balancing your stomach acids. Consumed before meal, this juice can make wonders.

<u>*Serves:*</u> *1*

<u>*Ready in:*</u> *5 minutes*

Ingredients:

½ Sweet Apple, halved
1/3 cup chopped Collard Greens
1 Mango, halved

Preparation:

1. Run all of the ingredients through your juicer, as instructed by your manufacturer.
2. Stir to combine.
3. Enjoy immediately!

Gingery Cabbage Pear Juice

This is probably one of the healthiest juices for your gut health that you will ever find. Enjoy before meals and balance your pH.

Serves: 1

Ready in: 5 minutes

Ingredients:

1/8 Red Cabbage
1 Pear, halved
1-inch piece of Ginger
¼ Cucumber
¼ Beet

Preparation:

1. Run all of the ingredients through your juices, following its instructions.
2. Stir to combine.
3. Consume immediately.
4. Enjoy!

Diluted Melon and Parsley Juice

Melon, parsley, cucumber, and water, make this light and super satisfying juice that will bring balance back to your stomach.

Serves: 1

Ready in: 5 minutes

Ingredients:

1/2 English Cucumber
½ cup Melon Chunks
A handful of Parsley
½ cup Coconut Water

Preparation:

1. Run the cucumber, melon, and parsley, through your juicer.
2. Pour the coconut water into the glass.
3. Stir to combine well.
4. Enjoy immediately!

Banana and Celery Juice

Seems like a strange combo, but this juice is super satisfying. Not to mention how alkalizing and healing it is.

Serves: 1

Ready in: 5 minutes

Ingredients:

1 Banana
2 Celery Stalks
½ Sweet Apple, halved
¼ cup Water
A small piece of Ginger

Preparation:

1. Juice the banana, celery, ginger, and apple, according to you juicer's instructions.
2. Pour the water into the glass.
3. Stir to combine.
4. Consume immediately and enjoy!

Watermelon and Basil Juice

Watermelon and holy basil are the starts of this recipe. Sweet, refreshing, and alkalizing, this juice is great at any time of the day.

<u>*Serves:*</u> 2

<u>*Ready in:*</u> *5 minutes*

Ingredients:

2 cups Watermelon Chunks
A handful of Holy Basil
½ Sweet Apple, halved

Preparation:

1. Run all of the ingredients through your juicer.
2. Stir to combine the mixture and pour into two serving glasses.
3. Consume immediately.
4. Enjoy!

Herbed Melony Juice

Melon, parsley, dill, and basil, are the stars of this recipe. Sweet and herbal, this juice will balance your pH and prepare your tummy for dinner.

<u>*Serves:*</u> *1*

<u>*Ready in:*</u> *5 minutes*

Ingredients:

1 cup Melon Chunks
1 tbsp Parsley
1 tbsp Dill
1 tbsp Basil

Preparation:

1. Juice all of the ingredients, and instructed by your manufacturer.
2. Stir to incorporate well.
3. Consume immediately.
4. Enjoy!

The Green Monster

Leafy greens, cucumber, avocado, apples, and celery, will restore your stomach balance and jumpstart the process of digestion.

<u>Serves:</u> 4

<u>Ready in:</u> 5 minutes

Ingredients:

1 cup Spinach
1 cup Kale Leaves
2 Sweet Apples
2 Celery Stalks
1 English Cucumber
½ Avocado
½ Banana

Preparation:

1. Cut the ingredients into juice-friendly pieces.
2. Juice them according to your juice's instructions.
3. Stir to combine and pour into 4 serving glasses.
4. Consume immediately or store in an airtight container in the fridge.
5. Enjoy!

Lettuce, Aloe Vera, and Avocado Juice

Packed with anti-inflammatory properties and highly alkalizing, this juice will relieve the symptoms of your upset gut.

Serves: 1

Ready in: 5 minutes

Ingredients:

1 Avocado
½ cup Lettuce
½ cup Aloe Vera Juice

Preparation:

1. Juice the avocado and lettuce following the instruction of your manufacturer.
2. Pour the aloe vera juice over and give it a good stir.
3. Consume right away.
4. Enjoy!

Papaya, Radish, and Cilantro Juice

Healthy, detoxifying, alkalizing, and extremely delicious, this juice will help you improve digestion if taken regularly.

Serves: 1

Ready in: 5 minutes

Ingredients:

½ cup Papaya Chunks
2 Radishes
1/3 cup Cilantro Leaves
1 Celery Stalk
½ Sweet Apple

Preparation:

1. Cut the ingredients into juice-manageable pieces.
2. Juice them according to your juicer's instructions.
3. Stir to combine well.
4. Serve and enjoy!

Blueberry Juice with Cucumber and Chard

Swiss chard, cucumber, blueberries, basil juiced together for a tummy-soothing purpose.

<u>*Serves:*</u> 1

<u>*Ready in:*</u> *5 minutes*

Ingredients:

2 Swiss Chard Leaves
¼ cup Blueberries
1 Cucumber
A handful of Basil

Preparation:

1. Chop the ingredients into juice-friendly pieces.
2. Run them through the juicer, following its instructions.
3. Stir to combine well and consume immediately.
4. Enjoy!

Spinach, Carrot, and Honeydew Juice

Alkalizing and anti-inflammatory, this juice will boost your tummy balance and help you digest your meals better.

Serves: 2

Ready in: 5 minutes

Ingredients:

1 cup Spinach
1 cup Honeydew Chunks
1 large Carrot
¼ Cucumber
1 Pear

Preparation:

1. Cut the ingredients into smaller chunks.
2. Run them through your juicer.
3. Stir the mixture to incorporate the juiced ingredients.
4. Divide among two serving glasses and consume right away.
5. Enjoy!

Orange Balancer

Mango, carrot, and cucumber join forces and create a powerful balancer that will prevent the after-meal heartburn.

Serves: 2

Ready in: 5 minutes

Ingredients:

2 Carrots
1 Cucumber
2 Mangos

Preparation:

1. Chop the ingredients into juicer-friendly chunks.
2. Juice them according to the juicer's instruction.
3. Stir to combine and divide among two serving glasses.
4. Enjoy immediately!

Peach and Ginger Juice

Fruity, sweet, and super delicious, this delightful juice will keep the heartburn and bay and restore your pH balance.

<u>*Serves:*</u> *1*

<u>*Ready in:*</u> *5 minutes*

Ingredients:

1 large Peach
1-inch Ginger Root
½ Pear
½ Sweet Apple
1 tbsp Dill

Preparation:

1. Run all of the ingredients through your juicer, as stated in its manual.
2. Stir the mixture to combine.
3. Serve immediately and enjoy!

All-Fruit Juice

Banana, raspberries, melon, papaya, and figs will fill your tummy before dinner, make you eat less, support digestion, and prevent the heartburn.

Serves: 2

Ready in: 5 minutes

Ingredients:

1 Banana
A handful of Fresh Raspberries
½ cup Papaya Chunks
½ cup Melon Chunks
2 Figs
½ cup Coconut Water

Preparation:

1. Run the fruits through your juicer.
2. Pour the coconut water over and give the mixture a good stir until it becomes fully incorporated.
3. Divide among two glasses.
4. Serve and enjoy!

Rainbow Booster

Containing all of the colors of the rainbow and a bunch of different vitamins, your health will surely benefit from this juice.

Serves: 2

Ready in: 5 minutes

Ingredients:

4 Strawberries
1 Mango
1 Sweet Apple
1 Banana
¼ Green Cabbage
¼ Cucumber
¼ cup Blueberries
1 Beetroot

Preparation:

1. Chop the ingredients into juicer-friendly slices.
2. Run them all through the juicer and stir to combine the mixture well.
3. Divide among 2 serving glasses.
4. Serve immediately and enjoy!

Golden Beet and Fig Juice

Cilantro, golden beet, fig, and melon make one delicious juice that will not only please your tummy, but balance it as well. If you want to, add a handful of spinach for a green juice.

Serves: 2

Ready in: 5 minutes

Ingredients:

1/3 cup Cilantro Leaves
1 ½ Golden Beets
2 Figs
1/2 cup Melon Chunks
¼ Cucumber

Preparation:

1. Run all of the ingredients through your juicer.
2. Stir to combine them well and divide among two serving glasses.
3. Serve immediately.
4. Enjoy!

Kale, Celery, and Cantaloupe Juice

The sweetness of the cantaloupe complements the sharp kale taste and the celery just wraps these two contrasts beautifully. Great before meals, but also super beneficial at any time of the day.

Serves: 1

Ready in: 5 minutes

Ingredients:

4 Kale Leaves
2 Celery Stalks
1 cup Cantaloupe Chunks

Preparation:

1. Juice the ingredients as stated in your juicer's manual.
2. Stir the mixture to combine well.
3. Serve immediately and enjoy.

Gingery Spinach, Fennel, and Mango Juice

The recipe name says it all. Packed with powerful alkalizing ingredients, this juice will nourish your stomach and balance its acids.

Serves: 2

Ready in: 5 minutes

Ingredients:

1-inch piece of Ginger
1 cup Spinach
A few Fennel Slices
2 Mangos
1 Sweet Apple
¼ Cucumber

Preparation:

1. Juice all of the ingredients following the juicer's instructions.
2. Stir to combine the mixture.
3. Pour into two serving glasses.
4. Consume immediately and enjoy!

Cold Afternoon Refreshments

If you want to refresh yourself with a delicious drink that will keep you hydrated and reduce the irritating symptoms of your acid reflux, then let this chapter show you amazingly delightful ways in which you can do that. Most of these recipes are water based and are great to consume in the afternoon, or 30 minutes before dinner to support proper gut function and heartburn relief.

Lavender Iced Drink

This recipe makes a lavender syrup that you can enjoy as an iced drink. Plus, this makes a great base for many mocktails.

Serves: 6

Ready in: 50 minutes

Ingredients:

½ cup Water
½ cup Sugar
1 tbsp dried Lavender
4 ½ cups Coconut Water
Ice Cubes, as needed

Preparation:

1. Combine the water and sugar in a saucepan over medium heat.
2. Bring to a boil and cook until the sugar is completely dissolved.
3. Remove from heat and stir in the raspberry.
4. Cover the saucepan and let the mixture sit for at least 30 minutes.
5. Strain and let the syrup cool for about 15 minutes.
6. Divide between 6 glasses.
7. Top with ice cubes and pour the coconut water over.
8. Stir and serve.
9. Enjoy!

Cucumber Water

Amazingly refreshing, delicious, and great for keeping the heartburn at bay, this coconut water will become your go-to refreshment.

<u>*Serves:*</u> 4

<u>*Ready in:*</u> *35 minutes*

Ingredients:

1 Basil Sprig
½ Cucumber, sliced
4 cups Water
Ice Cubes, as needed

Preparation:

1. Pour the water into a pitcher and add the remaining ingredients.
2. Give it a good stir
3. Let sit for about 30 minutes before enjoying.

Very Berry Flavored Water

Who doesn't like fresh berry flavors? This berry flavored water is a great way to curb your sweet cravings without adding any calories.

Serves: 4

Ready in: 35 minutes

Ingredients:

4 cups Water
4 Strawberries, halved
8 Raspberries
A handful of Blueberries
4 Blackberries

Preparation:

1. Combine all of the ingredients in a pitcher.
2. Place in your fridge and let sit for at least 30 minutes before serving.
3. Enjoy!

Chamomile and Ginger Iced Tea

Although this is great enjoyed as a warm tea, it is also delicious and satisfying when turned into an iced tea. Add some basil leaves if you want to add a more refreshing tone.

Serves: 4

Ready in: 30 minutes

Ingredients:

4 Chamomile Tea Bags
2-inch piece of Ginger Root, sliced
3 tbsp Maple Syrup
Ice Cubes, as needed
4 cups Boiling Water

Preparation:

1. Combine the chamomile, water, and ginger, in a saucepan.
2. Let steep for 5 minutes.
3. Discard the tea bags and let the mixture cool down, about 20 minutes or so.
4. Discard the ginger and whisk in the maple syrup.
5. Fill 4 glasses with ice cubes and pour the tea over.
6. Enjoy!

Melon Infused Water

Cantaloupe and honeydew are the starts of this recipe. This melon infused water will become your family's favorite. And the best part? It is extremely alkaline so there's an extra benefit for your tummy.

<u>*Serves:*</u> *4*

<u>*Ready in:*</u> *60 minutes*

Ingredients:

4 cups Water
½ cup Honeydew Chunks
½ cup Cantaloupe Chunks

Preparation:

1. Combine the water and fruit chunks in a pitcher.
2. Stir to combine and place in the fridge.
3. Let the water sit for at least 60 minutes to infuse the flavors.
4. Serve and enjoy!

Note: If you are impatient and cannot wait for an hour, poke the fruit chunks with a fork and serve after a couple of minutes over ice. The pokes will allow the fruit to release juices faster and infuse the water in a jiffy.

Ginger Ale

Ginger ale is a very popular refreshment, but the best part about this beverage is that it can actually help you reduce the acid reflux symptoms.

Serves: 8

Ready in: 30 minutes

Ingredients:

4 tbsp Maple Syrup
2 tbsp Brown Sugar
6 cups Water
1 ½ tbsp ground Ginger
1 tsp Cardamom Pods
Ice Cubes, as needed

Preparation:

1. Combine all of the ingredients in a saucepan.
2. Bring to a boil over medium heat and reduce to a simmer.
3. Cook for about 15 minutes.
4. Let the mixture sit for about an hour off the heat.
5. Strain through a fine mesh strainer.
6. Fill 8 cups with ice cubes and pour the ginger ale over.
7. Enjoy!

Rocking Ginger Apple Juice

Here is how you can easily make a gingery apple juice from scratch. Not only is this delicious, but it will also reduce the intensity of the acid reflux symptoms.

Serves: 4

Ready in: 15 minutes

Ingredients:

6 Sweet Apples
2-inch piece of Ginger, sliced
½ cup Coconut Water
Ice Cubes, as needed

Preparation:

1. Juice the apples according to the instructions of your juicer.
2. Pour into a pitcher and stir in the coconut water and ginger slices.
3. Fill 4 cups with ice cubes and pour the juice over.
4. Serve and enjoy!

Maple and Apple Iced Tea

Chamomile tea with maple and apple slices is turned into a refreshingly delicious iced tea that no one will be able to resist.

Serves: 4

Ready in: 15 minutes

Ingredients:

2 Chamomile Tea Bags
2 cups Boiling Water
1 cup Cold Apple Juice
1 cup Cold Water
8 Thin Sweet Apple Slices
2 tbsp Maple Syrup
Ice Cubes, as needed

Preparation:

1. Combine the tea bags and boiling water in a saucepan.
2. Cover and let steep for 5 minutes.
3. Allow to cool for about 5 minutes or so.
4. Pour into a pitcher along with your apple juice, water, and maple syrup.
5. Whisk to combine.
6. Stir in the apple slices and ice cubes.
7. Serve and enjoy!

Watermelon Water

This is perhaps one of the most refreshing drinks you will ever try. And that's not even the best part. The best part is that it is so alkalizing and healthy, that it will scare your heartburn away.

Serves: 8

Ready in: 60 minutes

Ingredients:

2 cups Watermelon Slices
8 cups Coconut Water
Ice Cubes, as needed

Preparation:

1. Combine the water and watermelon slices in a pitcher.
2. Refrigerate for at least 60 minutes before consuming.
3. Serve over ice.
4. Enjoy!

Note: Again, if you cannot wait 60 minutes, poke holes into the watermelon slices to speed up the process of infusing.

Nettle Iced Tea

Nettle, ginger, and blueberries, may not seem like a combination that you'd normally choose, but trust me, once you take a sip of this delightful iced tea, it will be your favorite one.

<u>*Serves:*</u> *2*

<u>*Ready in:*</u> *30 minutes*

Ingredients:

2 Nettle Tea Bags
1 Boiling Water
1 cup Cold Water
Ice Cubes, as needed
A handful of Blueberries

Preparation:

1. Combine the nettle and boiling water and let the tea steep for 5 minutes.
2. Let cool for about 10 minutes.
3. Pour into a pitcher and pour the cold water over.
4. Add blueberries and ice cubes and stir to combine.
5. Serve after 5 minutes.
6. Enjoy!

Gingery Iced Drink

Ginger syrup water, and ice. What more could you possibly want to cool yourself on a hot day? Besides, the ginger will not only give this drink an amazing flavor but it will also soothe your gut.

Serves: 3

Ready in: 60 minutes

Ingredients:

¼ cup Water
¼ cup Sugar
2-inch Ginger Root, sliced
2 cups Water
¼ cup Apple Syrup
Ice Cubes, as needed

Preparation:

1. Combine the water and sugar in a saucepan over medium heat.
2. Bring the mixture to a boil and cook for about a minute or two.
3. Remove from heat and stir in the ginger.
4. Cover and let steep for 30 minutes.
5. Discard the ginger and divide among 3 glasses.
6. Fill with ice cubes and pour the water over.
7. Top with apple juice and give the mixture a stir.
8. Serve and enjoy!

Vanilla and Pear Water

Vanilla and pear infused water? Yes, please. This combination is so divine that it will become a regular at your house.

Serves: 4

Ready in: 60 minutes

Ingredients:

1 Pear, sliced
1 Vanilla Bean
4 cups Water
Ice Cubes, as needed

Preparation:

1. Combine the water, pear, and vanilla bean, in your pitcher.
2. Place in the fridge and let sit for 60 minutes, or until infused.
3. Serve over ice.
4. Enjoy!

Fuji Apple & Cinnamon Iced Drink

Fuji apples combined with cinnamon and ice offer a delicious refreshment that is definitely approved by your acid reflux and GERD.

Serves: 4

Ready in: 15 minutes

Ingredients:

2 large Fuji Apples
4 cups Water
Ice Cubes, as needed
Pinch of Cinnamon

Preparation:

1. Peel, core, and chop the apples.
2. Place in your blender along with one cup of the water and cinnamon.
3. Blend until smooth.
4. Divide between 4 glasses.
5. Fill the glasses with ice cubes.
6. Top with water.
7. Serve and enjoy!

Apple Cider

Who says you cannot make your own apple cider at home? Follow these simple steps and see how easy it is.

Serves: 8

Ready in: 4 hours and 30 minutes

Ingredients:

8 Sweet Apples, peeled and quartered
16 cups Water
1 tbsp Cinnamon
½ cup Brown Sugar
1 tbsp All-Spice
Ice Cubes, as needed

Preparation:

1. Combine all of the ingredients, except the ice, in a large pot over medium heat.
2. Bring to a boil.
3. Let the mixture boil for about an hour.
4. Cover, reduce the hit, and cook for 2 more hours.
5. Remove from heat and let it cool completely.
6. Blend the mixture with a hand blender.
7. Run it through a strainer, until clean.
8. That is your cider.
9. Serve over ice.
10. Enjoy!

Hibiscus Iced Drink

You can also do this by using store-bought hibiscus syrup, but isn't it more fun to make your own?

Serves: 6

Ready in: 40 minutes

Ingredients:

1 Hibiscus Tea Bags
½ cup Water
½ cup Sugar
4 cups Water
Ice Cubes, as needed

Preparation:

1. Bring the water to a boil over medium heat.
2. Add the sugar and boil until it dissolves.
3. Add the hibiscus tea bag and remove from heat.
4. Cover the pan and let the mixture steep for 10 minutes.
5. Remove the teabag and let the syrup cool down.
6. Divide between 6 glasses.
7. Fill the glasses with ice cubes and pour the water over.
8. Serve and enjoy!

Peach Iced Tea

Chamomile and peach star in this super delicious iced tea recipe. You will never buy a peach iced tea ever again.

<u>*Serves:*</u> *4*

<u>*Ready in:*</u> *30 minutes*

Ingredients:

2 Chamomile Teabags
1 cup Boiling Water
4 Peaches
2 ½ cups Cold Water
Pinch of powdered Ginger
3 tbsp Maple Syrup
Ice Cubes, as needed

Preparation:

1. Combine the tea bags and water in a cup.
2. Let steep for 5 minutes.
3. Discard the tea bags.
4. Place the cold water in a pitcher and pour the tea over.
5. Juice the peaches following your juicer's instructions.
6. Pour into the pitcher.
7. Add ginger and maple syrup and whisk to combine.
8. Add the ice cubes and stir.
9. Serve and enjoy!

Blackberry & Rosemary Infused Water

It may seem strange, but blackberries and rosemary are a wonderful combination. Just trust me on this and give this recipe a try. I promise you will not regret it.

Serves: 4

Ready in: 60 minutes

Ingredients:

½ cup Blackberries
2 Rosemary Sprigs
4 cups Water
Ice Cubes, as needed

Preparation:

1. Combine the water, blackberries, and rosemary, in your pitcher.
2. Place in the fridge and let sit for about an hour.
3. Serve over ice.
4. Enjoy!

Rocking Aloe Vera Juice with Figs

Fig-flavored aloe vera juice on ice. Refreshment surely doesn't get better than this. Besides, the alkalizing properties of the figs combined with the heartburn-relieving power that aloe vera juice possesses is the perfect weapon to fight your acid reflux with.

<u>*Serves:*</u> 4

<u>*Ready in:*</u> *30 minutes*

Ingredients:

3 cups Aloe Vera Juice
½ cup Coconut Water
1 cup Ice Cubes
4 Figs, halved

Preparation:

1. Combine the aloe vera juice, coconut water, and figs, in your pitcher.
2. Place in the fridge and let sit there for 20 – 25 minutes.
3. Stir in the ice cubes and serve.
4. Do not forget to eat the figs after you drink the juice.
5. Enjoy!

Special Event Drinks

You don't have to be a party crasher just because alcohol is a total no-no for you. Make delicious and tummy-soothing mocktails instead, and enjoy the party with your fancy drinks.

Peach Cream "Soda"

Sweet, creamy, ice cold, fancy, and absolutely acid-reflux-approved, this peach cream "soda" is just the thing to serve at your next party.

Serves: 4

Ready in: 5 minutes

Ingredients:

½ cup Peach Syrup (that doesn't contain acidic ingredients)
¼ cup Heavy Cream
1 cup Coconut Water
Crushed Ice, about 2 cups

Preparation:

1. Divide the peach syrup between 4 glasses, about 2 tablespoons of syrup per glass.
2. Top the syrup with the crushed ice.
3. Slowly pour the coconut water (about ¼ cup of water per glass), until the glass is almost full.
4. Take a tablespoon of heavy cream and gently pour over the top.
5. Serve unmixed.
6. Enjoy!

Rosemary-Flavored Ginger & Apple Mimosas

Although this is a pretty simple drink to make, the rosemary sprig gives it an elegant touch that will wow your guests. And the best part? This mocktail is totally alkalizing.

Serves: 2

Ready in: 10 minutes

Ingredients:

½ cup Fresh Apple Juice
2 cups Coconut Water
2-inch piece of Ginger Root, sliced
10 Red Grapes
Crushed Ice, about 1 cup
2 Rosemary Sprigs

Preparation:

1. Pour the apple juice into 2 tall glasses.
2. Add a grape and some ginger into each glass.
3. Then, top with some of the ice.
4. Again, add a grape and some of the ginger.
5. Repeat until there are no more grapes and ginger pieces left.
6. Top with coconut water.
7. Garnish with a rosemary sprig.
8. Serve and enjoy!

Honeydew & Ginger "Spritzer"

Honeydew, ginger, and basil star in this amazingly delicious spritzer (without the fuzzy stuff, obviously) that will not only look fancy when served at your next event, but will also balance your tummy.

Serves: 3

Ready in: 5 minutes

Ingredients:

3 cups Honeydew Chunks
¼ cup Ginger Syrup
1 cup Coconut Water
1 ½ cups crushed Ice
A handful of Basil

Preparation:

1. Place the honeydew in your blender and blend until it becomes smooth and there are no more chunks left.
2. Add the coconut water and ginger syrup, and stir to combine well. Do NOT blend at this point.
3. Divide the ice among three serving glasses and pour the honeydew and ginger mixture over.
4. Top with basil leaves and serve.
5. Enjoy!

Mango Raspberry Ice Cream Shaker

Yes, this mocktail actually uses ice cream. That will not only take your party to a whole new level, but it will also satisfy your sweet and refreshing cravings without hurting your condition. How great is that?

Serves: 4

Ready in: 10 minutes

Ingredients:

1 Mango
1 cup frozen Raspberries
1 cup cold Coconut Water
4 Vanilla Ice Cream Scoops
1 cup Ice Cubes
12 Fresh or Frozen Raspberries

Preparation:

1. Place the mango, raspberries, and vanilla ice cream in your food processor or blender.
2. Pulse until smooth.
3. Divide the mixture among 4 serving glasses.
4. Add a couple of ice cubes to each glass.
5. Pour about ¼ cup of coconut water, or more if needed.
6. Give the mixture one gentle stir. Make sure not to mix everything up.
7. Top each mocktail with 3 raspberries.
8. Serve and enjoy!

Lavender Blueberry "Spritzer"

Known widely for its powerful healing properties, lavender is a great addition to this simple and yet super elegant mocktail.

<u>*Serves:*</u> 2

<u>*Ready in:*</u> *5 minutes*

Ingredients:

3 tbsp Lavender Syrup
2 tsp Blueberry Syrup
1 cup Coconut Water
A handful of Ice Cubes
A handful of blueberries
Fresh lavender, for garnishing

Preparation:

1. Place the ice cubes, lavender syrup, coconut water, and blackberry syrup, in a shaker.
2. Shake until the mixture becomes super cold.
3. Place the blueberries at the bottom of two champagne glasses.
4. Strain the lavender mixture and pour over the blueberries.
5. Garnish with some fresh lavender on top.
6. Enjoy!

Red & Orange Mocktail

This mango, watermelon, and coconut water cocktail will not only pack your stomach with powerful alkalizing properties but they will also super refresh and satisfy it as well.

Serves: 2

Ready in: 5 minutes

Ingredients:

1/3 cup Watermelon Chunks
1/3 cup Mango Chunks
2 tbsp Peach Syrup
½ cup crushed Ice
1 cup Coconut Water

Preparation:

1. Pour a tablespoon of peach syrup into the bottom of each tall glass.
2. Chop the watermelon chunks into even smaller pieces and top the syrup with them.
3. Place the crushed ice on top (this is important as it separates the red watermelon from the orange mango).
4. Pour the coconut water over.
5. Top with mango chunks.
6. Enjoy!

Cucumber "Mojito"

Who says you cannot serve mojito when you have frequent heartburn "attacks"? Ok, maybe every single doctor, but who says that you cannot make your own acid-reflux-friendly version? Try this one made with cucumbers and basil and see how overrated lime and mint are.

Serves: 6

Ready in: 60 minutes

Ingredients:

¼ cup Sugar
¼ cup Water
1/3 cup shredded Cucumber
½ cup Fresh Basil Leaves
Cucumber Water, as needed
Crushed Ice, as needed
6 unpeeled Cucumber Slices, for garnishing

Preparation:

1. Combine the water and sugar in a saucepan. Place over medium heat.
2. Bring to a boil and cook for about 1 minute. Remove from heat.
3. Stir in the shredded cucumber, immediately.
4. Cover the pan and let the mixture steep for about 30 minutes.
5. Strain it through a mesh sieve and let cool a bit.
6. Divide the cucumber syrup among 6 tall glasses.
7. Add the crushed ice and basil leaves.
8. Stir to combine everything well.
9. Pour enough cucumber water to fill the glasses. Do NOT stir at this point.
10. Garnish the glasses with a cucumber slice.
11. Serve and enjoy!

Peach Apple Shake

Peaches and apple juice star in this sweet and super uplifting non-alcoholic cocktail that works great for any occasion. This recipe uses sage leaves but you can garnish with something else if you are not a big sage fan.

Serves: 2

Ready in: 10 minutes

Ingredients:

1 cup Peach Chunks
¼ cup Water
1 cup Apple Juice (made with sweet apples)
½ cup Ice
4 Sage Leaves

Preparation:

1. Combine the water and peach chunks in your blender.
2. Blend until the mixture becomes smooth and there are no more chunks left.
3. Transfer to a shaker.
4. Add the ice and apple juice and shake until it becomes super cold.
5. Pour into 2 fancy glasses (do NOT strain).
6. Top with two sage leaves.
7. Enjoy!

Sugary Peach Apple Cider

Apple cider may be great to cool down in your backyard on a hot summer afternoon, but it isn't the fanciest drink to serve on its own. But, combine it with cinnamon sugar and peach juice and you've got yourself a winning combination.

<u>Serves:</u> 2

<u>Ready in:</u> 5 minutes

Ingredients:

1/2 cup Apple Cider
1 cup Peach Chunks
½ cup Water
2 tbsp Cinnamon Sugar
½ cup Ice Cubes
4 thin Peach Slices

Preparation:

1. Brush the edges of two martini glasses with some apple cider and rim them with cinnamon sugar.
2. Place the peach chunks and water in your blender and blend until smooth.
3. Transfer to a shaker along with the apple cider and ice.
4. Shake the mixture well, until really cold.
5. Divide the peach slices among the glasses.
6. Strain the peach and apple cider mixture and pour over the peach.
7. Serve and enjoy!

Grilled Papaya & Pear Mocktail

Papaya and pear turns out to be a divine combination. And a one that will lower your acid reflux symptoms.

<u>*Serves:*</u> *4*

<u>*Ready in:*</u> *5 minutes*

Ingredients:

1 cup Papaya Slices
2 tbsp Maple Syrup
1 cup Pear Chunks
¼ tsp Cinnamon
1 ½ cups Coconut Water
A handful of Ice Cubes

Preparation:

1. Preheat your grill to medium.
2. In a small bowl, combine the maple syrup and cinnamon.
3. Brush the mixture over the papaya.
4. Place the papaya slices on the preheated grill and grill until slightly blackened.
5. Reserve 4 Papaya sliced and transfer the rest of them to your blender.
6. Add the pear chunks, coconut water, and ice cubes to the blender.
7. Blend until smooth.
8. Divide between 4 glasses. Do not worry about the black spots, because they should be visible. That is what makes this recipe unique and give this mocktail a charred flavor.
9. Garnish the glasses with the reserved papaya slices.
10. Serve and enjoy!

A Different Shirley Temple

Ginger ale, peach syrup, and candied ginger. How amazing does that sound? Serve this at your next event and watch it disappear in no time.

<u>Serves:</u> 2

<u>Ready in:</u> 5 minutes

Ingredients:

4 tbsp Peach Syrup
2 cups Ginger Ale
½ cup Ice Cubes
2 tbsp Candied Ginger

Preparation:

1. Brush the edges of two glasses with some peach syrup and rim them with candied ginger. The syrup will help the candied ginger stick to the glass.
2. Combine the rest of the ingredients in a shaker and shake until cold.
3. Strain and pour into the glasses.
4. Enjoy!

Watermelon Ginger Cooler

Clear and super delicious, this mocktail will relieve your from the irritating heartburn almost instantly. You can serve this with ice cubes instead, but the crushed ice gives it a more elegant look.

<u>*Serves:*</u> *2*

<u>*Ready in:*</u> *5 minutes*

Ingredients:

1 ½ cup Watermelon Chunks
1/2 cup Apple Juice (made with sweet apples)
½ cup Water
1-inch Ginger Root, sliced very thinly
Crushed Ice, as needed

Preparation:

1. Place the watermelon, apple juice, and water, in a blender.
2. Blend until really smooth.
3. Strain the mixture well through a fine mesh sieve, until clear.
4. Divide the ice between two glasses and pour the watermelon mixture over.
5. Add the ginger slices and mix to combine.
6. Serve and enjoy!

Virgin Mai Tai

Apple cider, ginger, and maple syrup are the stars of this virgin version of Mai Tai. This recipe uses orgeat syrup that is found in the classic Mai Tai, but if you cannot find it, you can substitute it with ginger syrup and a drop of Almond extract.

<u>*Serves:*</u> *2*

<u>*Ready in:*</u> *5 minutes*

Ingredients:

1 cup Apple Cider
8 Ginger Slices
1 ounce Maple Syrup
1 ounce Orgeat (Almond Syrup)
Ice Cubes, as needed
Crushed Ice, as needed

Preparation:

1. In a shaker, combine the apple cider, maple syrup, orgeat, and some ice cubes.
2. Shake until cold and well combined.
3. Fill two double rocks glasses with crushed ice.
4. Strain the mocktail and pour over the crushed ice.
5. Add ginger and stir to combine.
6. Enjoy!

Cucumber Fig Cooler

Figs and cucumbers give this ice-cold mocktail a delicious taste and rich flavor that will not only satisfy your tummy, but also balance the pH levels.

Serves: 2

Ready in: 5 minutes

Ingredients:

1 cup chopped Figs
1 cup Water
¼ Cucumber, chopped
8 Cucumber Slices
½ cup Ice Cubes

Preparation:

1. Place the cucumber, figs, and water in your blender.
2. Pulse until smooth.
3. Transfer the mixture to a shaker and add the ice.
4. Shake well until cool.
5. Divide the mixture among two glasses.
6. Add 4 cucumber slices to each glass.
7. Serve and enjoy!

Tropical Cheesecake Mocktail

Cream cheese in a cocktail? It may sound like a strange combo but once you take a sip of this delightfully satisfying mocktail, you will see how incredibly tasty it is. And the best part? It is packed with alkalizing properties that will soothe your symptoms.

Serves: 2

Ready in: 5 minutes

Ingredients:

1 tbsp Cream Cheese
1 tbsp Heavy Cream
½ cup Papaya Chunks
1/3 cup Mango Chunks
¼ cup Almond Milk
2/3 cup Water
1 tbsp Maple Syrup

½ cup Ice Cubes
Crushed Ice, as needed

Preparation:

1. Place the papaya and mango chunks in your food processor and pulse until pureed.
2. Place the puree in a shaker along with the cream cheese, heavy cream, maple syrup, and ice cubes.
3. Shake the mixture well until really cold and the heavy cream becomes somewhat whipped.
4. Fill two glasses with crushed ice and divide the mixture between them.
5. Pour the almond milk on top. Make sure NOT to mix.
6. Enjoy!

Coconut Cream Punch

Fruit juice, coconut cream, and heavy cream, give this cocktail a deliciously creamy texture that is hard to resist.

<u>*Serves:*</u> *2*

<u>*Ready in:*</u> *5 minutes*

Ingredients:

2 ounces Coconut Cream
2 ounces Heavy Cream
1 cup Fresh Fruit Juice by your choice (non-acidic)
Pinch of Cinnamon, for garnish
Ice Cubes

Preparation:

1. Place the coconut cream, heavy cream, fruit juice and a handful of ice cubes, in a shaker.
2. Shake well until cold and well combined.
3. Divide between two glasses.
4. Sprinkle with some cinnamon on top.
5. Serve and enjoy!

Appletini

Apple mocktail in a martini glass spiced up with some ginger and cinnamon. Not only yummy but heartburn relieving as well.

<u>*Serves:*</u> *3*

<u>*Ready in:*</u> *5 minutes*

Ingredients:

1 cup Apple Juice (made with sweet apples)
1 tbsp Ginger Syrup
½ cup Cucumber Water
½ cup Sweet Apple Chunks
Pinch of Cinnamon
6 Ginger Slices

Preparation:

1. Place the apple chunks in a food processor and pulse until pureed.
2. Transfer to a shaker.
3. Add the apple juice, cucumber water, ginger syrup, cinnamon, and ice.
4. Shake well until combined and ice cold.
5. Strain the mixture and pour into martini glasses.
6. Stir two slices of ginger into each appletini.
7. Serve immediately and enjoy!

Creamy Nectarine Breeze

Although technically a smoothie, the elegance of this non-alcoholic drink is what makes it a great mocktail that can be served on any special event.

Serves: 3

Ready in: 5 minutes

Ingredients:

1 cup chopped Nectarines
½ cup Apple Juice (made with sweet apples)
3 ounces Coconut Milk
3 ounces Almond Milk
3 Thin Coconut Slices
Crushed Ice, as needed

Preparation:

1. Place the nectarines, apple juice, almond milk, and coconut milk, in your blender.
2. Blend the mixture until smooth.
3. Fill three glasses with crushed ice.
4. Pour the creamy nectarine mixture over.
5. Garnish each of the glasses with a coconut slice.
6. Serve immediately and enjoy!

Raspberry, Apple & Ginger Cooler

Sweet, berry-flavored, and rich in gingery aroma, this mocktail is one of the most delicious heartburn-friendly cocktails that you will ever find.

Serves: 1

Ready in: 5 minutes

Ingredients:

5 Raspberries, halved
1-inch Ginger Root, minced
1 tbsp Maple Syrup
3 ounces Apple Juice (made with sweet apples as sour ones can aggravate your condition)
2 ounces Ginger Ale
Ice Cubes, as needed

Preparation:

1. Place the ice cubes, raspberries, ginger, and maple syrup, in a shaker.
2. Muddle well.
3. Add the apple juice and shake until the mixture is well combined and ice cold.
4. Fill a glass with a few ice cubes.
5. Strain the cocktail well and pour into the glass.
6. Top with the Ginger Ale, but do not mix.
7. Serve and enjoy!

Watermelon Bloody Meru

OK, this isn't technically a Bloody Meru, but the rich red color and creamy texture give us the right to call it so. Watermelon and cucumber drink with a celery stick. Yummy!

Serves: 4

Ready in: 5 minutes

Ingredients:

3 cups Watermelon Chunks
½ Cucumber, chopped
½ cup Apple Juice (made with sweet apples)
2 Celery Sticks, halved
Crushed Ice, as needed

Preparation:

1. Place the watermelon, cucumber, and apple juice in your blender.
2. Blend until the mixture becomes smooth.
3. Fill 4 glasses with crushed ice and pour the mixture over.
4. Place a celery stick half into each glass.
5. Serve and enjoy!

Lavender & Strawberry Mocktail

Lavender and strawberry mocktail with coconut water and basil leaves. Although you can substitute the basil leaves with other herbs, I highly suggest them as they give this drink a fresh note that wraps everything up beautifully.

Serves: 2

Ready in: 5 minutes

Ingredients:

2 tbsp Lavender Syrup
2 tbsp Strawberry Syrup, made with heartburn-friendly ingredients only
1 cup Coconut Water
10 Basil Leaves
Some Fresh Lavender, for garnish
Ice Cubes, about ½ cup

Preparation:

1. Place the lavender syrup, strawberry syrup, ice, and half of the coconut water, in a shaker.
2. Shake until the mixture is well combined and ice cold.
3. Place the basil leaves at the top of two double rock glasses.
4. Pour the mixture over.
5. Top with the remaining coconut water.
6. Garnish with some lavender flowers on top.
7. Serve and enjoy!

Mango & Maple Punch

Mango, apple juice, passion fruit, and maple syrup are the main ingredients in this lovely mocktail that will not only not aggravate your symptoms, but they can also relieve the heartburn.

Serves: 3

Ready in: 5 minutes

Ingredients:

1 cup Mango Chunks
2/3 cup Apple Juice (made with sweet apples, not sour ones)
2 tbsp Maple Syrup
1/3 cup Passion Fruit Juice
Ice Cubes, as needed
4 Edible Flowers, for garnish

Preparation:

1. Place the mango chunks in a food processor and pulse until pureed.
2. Transfer to a shaker along with the maple syrup, passion fruit juice, and ice.
3. Shake well until ice cold.
4. Strain the mixture and pour into 3 glasses.
5. Top with the apple juice and give the punch a stir to combine.
6. Garnish the glasses with edible flowers.
7. Serve and enjoy!

Creamy Fennel Cooler

Fennel syrup, heavy cream, and coconut water, are surprisingly a great combo. Do not skip the almond syrup as that's what gives this mocktail a warming tone.

<u>Serves:</u> 6

<u>Ready in:</u> 60 minutes

Ingredients:

¼ cup Water
¼ cup Sugar
¼ Fennel Bulb, sliced
1 1/2 cup Coconut Water
6 tbsp Heavy Cream
3 tbsp Almond Syrup
Crushed Ice, as needed
6 Fennel Fronds

Preparation:

1. Combine the water and sugar in a saucepan over medium heat.
2. Bring the mixture to a boil and let it boil for a minute or so.
3. Remove from heat and stir in the fennel.
4. Cover the pan and let steep for about 30 minutes.
5. Discard the fennel and let cool a bit.
6. Divide the fennel syrup between 6 glasses.
7. Top with ½ tbsp of the almond syrup.
8. Fill the glasses with crushed ice and pour the coconut water over.
9. Stir to combine.
10. Pour 1 tbsp of heavy cream over but do NOT mix at this point.
11. Gently stick a fennel ford into each glass, making sure not to mix the mocktail.
12. Serve and enjoy!

Wassail-Like Mocktail

For the final mocktail recipe, I decided to go with this warm beverage. This mockail is spiced up with ginger, allspice, and cloves, but if you are by any chance aggravated by cloves or allspice, make sure to omit them. Adding cinnamon to the mixture should be just as delicious. Enjoy!

Serves: 8

Ready in: 55 minutes

Ingredients:

4-inch Ginger Root, sliced
2 tsp Whole Cloves
2 tsp Allspice Berries
1 cup juiced Papaya
½ gallon Apple Cider
1 cup juiced Mango
2 tbsp Maple Syrup
½ Apple, thinly sliced

Preparation:

1. Cut a 10-inch cheesecloth piece and add the spices to it.
2. Tie them together.
3. Combine the apple cider and juices in a saucepan and place the spice packet in it.
4. Bring the mixture to a simmer.
5. Cook for about 35 minutes, but do NOT bring to a boil.
6. Remove from heat and whisk in the maple syrup.
7. Pour into 8 glasses and add an apple slice inside.
8. Serve warm and enjoy!

<u>Warming & Relieving Tea</u>

Warming tea recipes and blends that can help you fight your vexing condition. Most of these recipes are really simple and easy to make, but there are also some for the more experiences tea blenders that use not-so-common ingredients.

Great for any time of the day!

Simple Ginger Tea

If you find this too bland for your taste, feel free to flavor it up with some maple syrup, or even add a splash of milk to it (yes, almond and coconut milk will both work fine). Great for soothing your tummy.

Serves: 1

Ready in: 5 minutes

Ingredients:

1 cup of Boiling Water
2-inch piece of Ginger Root

Preparation:

1. Peel and slice your ginger.
2. Place it in a teacup and pour the boiling water over.
3. Let it steep for 5 minutes.
4. Enjoy!

Note: There is no need to discard the ginger – the longer it steeps the richer the flavor and the healthier the tea for your acid reflux.

Licorice Root Tea

The strong taste of this tea is really not for everyone, however, since it can basically do wonders for your gut, I highly suggest to consume this tea on regular basis. Sweeten it up with maple syrup or add a more pleasing touch such as ground cinnamon to it.

<u>*Serves:*</u> *3*

<u>*Ready in:*</u> *10 minutes*

Ingredients:

3 cups Boiling Water
1-inch Licorice Root

Preparation:

1. Cut the licorice root in half and place it on a piece of parchment paper.
2. Top with another piece of parchment paper and pound it with a meat pounder until chunky.
3. Transfer to a mortar and grind the root well.
4. Add about ½ teaspoon to a mesh tea steeper, or tie it into a bundle in a small piece of cheesecloth.
5. Pour the boiling water over and enjoy after 5 minutes.

Note: Keep in mind that to get the best results here, you need to have a least ½ teaspoon of ground licorice root. If you don't have that from an inch of root, decrease the servings to 2 or grind some more licorice.

Sage and Lavender Tea

This tea is not only rich in pleasant flavor, but it also tastes great. Warm your stomach and relieve your acid reflux symptoms with a cup of this tea.

Serves: 2

Ready in: 7 minutes

Ingredients:

4 dried Sage Leaves
1 tbsp dried Lavender
2 cups Boiling Water

Preparation:

1. Place the sage and lavender in your mortar.
2. Grind it until finely ground.
3. Cut two 10-inch squares of cheesecloth and divide the mixture among them.
4. Tie them into bundles and place each bundle in a teacup.
5. Pour the boiling water over and let steep for 5 minutes.
6. Serve and enjoy!

Apple and Cinnamon Tea

Here is something you might not have known before – dried fruits make a delicious tea. When you get bored of your traditional herbal tea, make this recipe. I guarantee that you will be satisfied.

Serves: 4

Ready in: 10 minutes

Ingredients:

1 ½ cups dried Sweet Apple sliced
1 Cinnamon Stick
4 cups Water
2 tbsp Maple Syrup

Preparation:

1. Place the water in a saucepan and bring to a boil.
2. Remove from heat immediately and stir in the apple and cinnamon.
3. Cover the pan and let it steep for at least 5 minutes.
4. Strain the mixture and whisk in the maple syrup.
5. Serve immediately and enjoy!

Simple Chamomile Tea

We know that chamomile tea is very soothing, but what you might not have known is that these magical flowers can also relieve your acid reflux symptoms. This is probably the best tea to enjoy at night. A good night's sleep is an added bonus.

Serves: 1

Ready in: 5 minutes

Ingredients:

1 tsp dried Chamomile Flowers
1 cup Boiling Water

Preparation:

1. Place the chamomile flowers in your tea mash strain or time them into a bundle in a small piece of cheesecloth.
2. Place in a teacup.
3. Pour the boiling water over.
4. Let the chamomile steep for 5 minutes.
5. Enjoy immediately!

After Meal Tea

Chamomile tea and licorice root are perfect to consume after meal (not right after though, about 30 minutes or so after your meal).

Serves: 4-5

Ready in: 7 minutes

Ingredients:

1 tsp dried and ground Licorice Root
4 tsp dried Chamomile
4-5 cups Boiling Water

Preparation:

1. Combine the licorice root and chamomile in a small bowl.
2. Divide between 4 or 5 10-inch cheesecloth pieces and tie them into bundles.
3. Place in teacups and pour the boiling over water.
4. Consume after 5 minutes.
5. Enjoy!

Note: You don't have to serve the tea immediately. If you tie the herbs into bundles, you can easily store the cheesecloth tea bags and enjoy later.

Immune-Boosting Tea

Not only will this tea help you keep the heartburn at bay, but it will also improve your overall immune system and keep the flu away from you.

Serves: 4

Ready in: 10 minutes

Ingredients:

4 Sage Leaves
1 tsp dried ground Hibiscus
1 tsp dried Elderflowers
1 tsp dried Calendula Flowers
4 cups Boiling Water

Preparation:

1. Place all of the herbs in your mortar.
2. Grind until finely ground and powder-like.
3. Divide between 4 cheesecloth pieces and tie into bundles. Alternatively, you can place a teaspoon of the mixture into a tea mesh strainer.
4. Place into teacups and pour the boiling water over.
5. Serve after 5 minutes.
6. Enjoy!

Nettle Tea

Nettle is one of the healthiest herbs on the planet, so it is pretty obvious that you can only benefit from this tea. However, this is also great for your special condition as it will soothe your gut and reduce the symptoms of your irritating condition.

Serves: 1

Ready in: 5 minutes

Ingredients:

5 dried Nettle Leaves
1 cup Boiling Water

Preparation:

1. Place the nettle leaves in a teacup.
2. Pour the boiling water over.
3. Let it steep for 5 minutes.
4. Enjoy!

Note: You can also grind the nettle and tie them into a cheesecloth bundle. The effect will be the same.

Roasted Barley Cinnamon Tea

Roasted barley can be bought in pretty much all Japanese food stores as this is the most famous Japanese after-meal tea. I added cinnamon for extra flavor and added health benefits.

Serves: 2

Ready in: 10 minutes

Ingredients:

2 teabags Roasted Barley Tea
1 tsp Cinnamon Chips
2 cups Water

Preparation:

1. Pour the water into a saucepan. Bring it to a boil over medium heat. Or you can simply use a kettle and pour boiling water into a saucepan.
2. Turn the heat off and add the cinnamon chips and roasted barley tea.
3. Cover the pan and let the mixture sit for 5 minutes.
4. Strain and pour into 2 cups.
5. Serve immediately.
6. Enjoy!

Rooibos & Apple Tea

Red bush tea (rooibos) is packed with tons of detoxifying properties that can help you restore the balance in your tummy. The apple is a delicious bonus that your health will also benefit from.

<u>*Serves:*</u> *1*

<u>*Ready in:*</u> *5 minutes*

Ingredients:

1 teabag Rooibos Tea
2 tsp dried Sweet Apple Chips
1 cup Boiling Water

Preparation:

1. Combine all of the ingredients in a teacup.
2. Let it steep for 5 minutes.
3. Remove the tea bag and apple chips.
4. Enjoy immediately!

Apple Cider & Ginger Tea

Warm apple cider and fresh ginger combine forces to knock down your acid reflux symptoms. A warming and very pleasing cup of tea.

Serves: 1

Ready in: 10 minutes

Ingredients:

½ cup Apple Cider
½ cup Water
1-inch Piece of Ginger, sliced

Preparation:

1. Place the water in a saucepan over medium heat and bring it to a boil.
2. Add the apple cider and cook until just until it starts to boil. Remove when the first bubbles appear.
3. Add the ginger and let the mixture sit for about 5 minutes or so.
4. Pour the tea into a teacup, unstrained.
5. Enjoy immediately.

Soothing Fennel Tea

Chamomile, ginger, and fennel seeds make one soothing cup of tea. Add some maple syrup to sweeten it up and enjoy!

Serves: 1

Ready in: 7 minutes

Ingredients:

1 tsp dried Chamomile Flowers
6 Ginger Slices
1/3 tsp Fennel Seeds
1 cup Boiling Water

Preparation:

1. Add the chamomile, ginger, and fennel, to a small piece of cheesecloth.
2. Tie into a bundle and place in a teacup.
3. Pour the water over.
4. Let it steep for at least 5 minutes.
5. Enjoy immediately!

Detox Tea

Nettle, dandelion, cloves, and juniper berries are combined together to support proper gut function and purge the toxins away from your body. If you are sensitive to some of these ingredients, substitute with chamomile tea.

Serves: 4

Ready in: 7 minutes

Ingredients:

1 tsp Cloves
1 tsp dried ground Nettle
1 tsp dried Dandelion Root
1 tsp Juniper Berries
4 cups Boiling Water

Preparation:

1. Cut a 10-inch piece of ginger and place the cloves, nettle, dandelion, and juniper on it.
2. Tie them into a bundle and place in a saucepan.
3. Pour the boiling water over and cover the pan.
4. Let steep for 5 minutes.
5. Pour into 4 glasses and enjoy!

Comfort Tea

If you like buying comfort tea blends, then you will absolutely love this combination. Besides being comforting, this tea blend will also knock down the heartburn.

<u>*Serves:*</u> *4*

<u>*Ready in:*</u> *10 minutes*

Ingredients:

1 ¼ tsp dried ground Licorice Root
1 tsp dried Chamomile
½ tsp dried ground Basil
½ tsp Fennel Seeds
4 cups Boiling Water

Preparation:

1. Cut 4 small squares of cheesecloth.
2. Combine the herbs in a small bowl and divide between the cheesecloth.
3. Tie them into bundles and place in teacups.
4. Pour the boiling water over and let steep for 5 minutes.
5. Consume immediately!

The Ultimate Heartburn Reliever

Although some of these ingredients are not that easy to find, their powerful properties make the search to be worthwhile. A few sips of this tea will knock down your heartburn almost instantly.

Serves: 6

Ready in: 10 minutes

Ingredients:

1 tsp dried Elderberry
1 tsp Norwegian Angelica
1 tsp Iceland Moss
½ tsp Juniper Berries
1 tsp Yellow Gentian
1 tsp dried Chamomile
1 tsp dried Wormwood
6 cups Boiling Water

Preparation:

1. Make 6 small squares out of a cheesecloth.
2. Combine all of the herbs in a small bowl and divide the mixture among the cheesecloth pieces.
3. Tie them into bundles and place each of them in a teacup.
4. Pour a cup of boiling tea over and let sit for 5 minutes.
5. Consume immediately.
6. Enjoy!

Rose Hip, Nettle, and Cinnamon Tea

This nourishing tea will not only boost your iron and vitamin C content, but it will also soothe your upset gut.

<u>Serves:</u> 4

<u>Ready in:</u> 10 minutes

Ingredients:

1 tsp Cinnamon Chips
2 tsp dried and ground Nettle
2 tsp dried and ground Rose Hips
4 cups Boiling Water

Preparation:

1. Cut 4 squares out of a cheesecloth.
2. Combine all of the ingredients in a bowl and divide among the squares, equally.
3. Tie them into bundles and place in teacups.
4. Pour with boiling water.
5. Let steep or 5 minutes.
6. Consume immediately and enjoy!

Harmony Tea

To restore not only the mental but the harmony and balance of your body as well, try this tea. Your upset stomach will thank you later.

Serves: 4

Ready in: 7 minutes

Ingredients:

1 tsp ground minced Ginger
1 tsp Chaste Tree Berries
½ tsp dried Oatstraw
½ tsp Blessed Thistle
2 tsp dried Chamomile
4 cups Boiling Water

Preparation:

1. Cut a square out of cheesecloth, large enough to fit all of the herbs.
2. Tie into a bundle and place in a saucepan.
3. Pour the water over.
4. Cover the saucepan and let the mixture steep for 5 minutes.
5. Remove the cheesecloth and pour into 4 teacups.
6. Enjoy immediately!

Spring Tea

Nourishing and satisfying, this warming tea will uplift your mood and reduce the acid reflux symptoms.

Serves: 1

Ready in: 7 minutes

Ingredients:

¼ tsp ground Dandelion Root
1/2 tsp minced Ginger
½ tsp dried Red Clover
¼ tsp dried Licorice Root
1 cup of Boiling Water

Preparation:

1. Combine all of the ingredients in a tea mesh strainer or place on a piece of cheesecloth and tie into a bundle.
2. Place in a teacup and pour the boiling water over.
3. Steep for 5 minutes.
4. Enjoy immediately.

Conclusion

Now that you know what you have to do in order to battle acid reflux while pleasing your taste buds, the next step is to turn your blender/juicer on, grab some healthy and yummy ingredients, and start enjoying these delightful beverages.

Once you begin incorporating highly alkalizing foods into your diet you will see that the heartburn will become a rarer occurrence, and your acid reflux symptoms will be significantly reduced. And all thanks to these heartburn-friendly beverages.

Love a good challenge? I dare you to try them all.

If you enjoyed the book, please leave a review on Amazon! Thanks ☺

Some design elements of the book cover were created by Freepik (http://www.freepik.com)

Made in United States
North Haven, CT
10 December 2023

45452615R00075